6 Organic Douches

T.R. Hodges

"It's your body. Make it a healthy one"

"Make the choice, own your health, use organic remedies"

6 Organic Douches

Text Copyright© 2016 T.R. Hodges

For more great tips on living an organic, low cost lifestyle, visit

www.digitalquill.top

This book is dedicated to the ladies that want to renew their health by working with nature to restore balance. Only in working with the natural resources that God has so richly given us can we hope to successfully balance the marvelous creation known as the body.

Table of Contents

Chapter 1

Douching has been a long standing tradition that gives females a fresh feeling in their intimate parts. It can be traced back as far as the year 1766 and is attributed to the Italian language meaning 'conduit pipe' and 'pour by drops'.

In English, a douche is traditionally known as a liquid that is streamed into the vaginal cavity. The liquid being streamed can vary ingredient-wise. The douche may be water-based with additional ingredients such as vinegar or tea tree oil which is the healthiest type of douche or it may be chemical-based douche such as the ones sold over the counter.

At one point, there were douches available over the counter, however, these did not always work well. They were designed to be a rinse for the vaginal area and not for actual medicinal purposes. Some included chemical scents that were touted to cover unpleasant feminine odor, but did nothing to actually remedy the cause of the odor. These chemicals, in some cases, exacerbated the problem making it worse and requiring medical care.

Not all douches are equal. Some work better than others according to any issues that may be present in the body and the body's chemistry. The best douches are the organic, natural ones that work with the body's chemistry to encourage and produce a healthy environment while killing foreign agents that cause irritation and infection. While douching can bring harmony to the intimate parts of the body, it is, as with everything, to be done in moderation.

It is possible to over-douche. The vagina is self-lubricating and self-balancing. It has its own natural balance that includes naturally occurring flora much like the intestinal tract. The idea behind douching is to gently restore balance and healthy lubrication. However, the balance can be upset in several ways: food, chemicals, disease and swimming.

FOOD:

The old adage 'you are what you eat' is very true. Food can balance or unbalance the body. Bad food can cause imbalances throughout the body which manifest more predominantly in one area or another, with some symptoms being more overt than others.

Take for example sugar. Sugar tastes good. It makes coffee sweeter, cookies more appealing and it is a *must* have for chocolate. A healthy body can process small amounts of sugar effectively, but when the body is subjected to large quantities, it creates a heavy imbalance such as a yeast infection.

Yeast feeds on sugar and when the body is overwhelmed and can no longer balance itself, an overabundance of yeast ravages the body. It resides in the brain, the intestines, the bowels, the sexual parts, the feet, the nails, the skin and even the scalp.

Yeast is not gender specific. It affects males as well as females. Women tend to have yeast symptoms in the vaginal area whereas men tend to have symptoms such as jock itch, foot fungus, nail fungus and loss of hair on the scalp.

The scary thing about yeast is that the body virtually has to be overrun internally before there are external symptoms such as fatigue, mental acuity loss, flatulence, nail loss and irritable bowels.

The good news is it is easy to kill yeast internally and externally with natural, organic substances and without the use of antibiotics which the body tends to build an immunity to.

CHEMICALS:
Chemicals can also cause imbalances in the body. Many body products such as body washes, deodorants and shampoos have harmful chemicals in them that are hormone disrupters. These usually affect women more severely than men as women have a hormonal cycle that is much more complex than men's. These chemicals can be very destructive to girls who have not yet reached puberty and those just entering puberty because the cycle initiated in a pre-pubescent female needs normal hormonal activity to successfully make the transition into womanhood.

A lot of hormones are needed at the correct levels to complete this phase and set the body up for motherhood. These hormone disrupting products, many that are marketed towards young girls, are virtually destroying their bodies' ability to successfully complete the puberty phase. They wreak havoc on a young body not designed to handle chemicals and make harmful imbalances that can affect them for life.

These imbalances from chemicals can cause the vaginal tissues to be undermined, making it weak to fight off infections, unable to balance itself and altering the chemical makeup so that it is more acidic than basic. When body chemistry is more acidic than basic, this sets the environment for cancer.

DISEASE:
Cancer is a disease that lives in an altered chemical environment in the body. Other diseases also affect the vaginal area such as Herpes, AIDS and Syphilis. Some diseases produce a direct symptom in the vaginal area while others have a more ambiguous effect. But once imbalance is present in the body, the entire body is affected and not just a single area.

For instance, yeast may be the single cause, but it produces imbalances in different parts of the body which have numerous manifested symptoms. When the brain is overrun with yeast, the mind is cloudy, it is hard to think and memory is reduced. When yeast is present in the hands or feet, nail fungus occurs which can cause fingernail or toenail loss. When the scalp is yeast ridden, hair thinning and hair loss occur. When bowels are saturated with yeast, irritable bowels, flatulence and irregular stool creation call occur. All of these symptoms and more can be manifested in a single person but the causal factor is one thing: yeast. Kill the yeast, stop eating the foods that cause yeast overabundance and the body will be well on its way to rebalancing itself.

The body is largely a self-containing, self-correcting system. When one part of the body is out of balance, the rest of the body works to reset that balance. The body works 24/7, continuously trying to achieve and maintain proper balance. What is amazing is that we don't consciously know that this is going on every minute of every day. The body is hardwired to fix itself. Can you imagine if we had to think about healing our bodies every time something attacked it? We wouldn't have a life! We couldn't sleep because we would be overrun. We couldn't do anything but focus our energy on healing.

Fortunately, we don't have to think about healing our bodies because our bodies do the work for us without us having to think about it. It is automatic. It is a beautiful. It enables us to have a life.

When the body is mostly healthy, it can achieve balance within itself, not needing outside assistance or special consideration. It will ebb and flow as it needs to fight foreign invaders or readjust to outside factors such as poor air quality or a sunburn. But when the body is fighting too many battles on too many fronts, it becomes overwhelmed and can't right itself.

When the body is overwhelmed, symptoms are more pronounced internally and/or externally. It is easy to see there is an imbalance and that a fix is needed. When symptoms appear, outside intervention is required to rebalance the body. While douching may help reset the internal flora balance, it may be indicative of an underlying cause which needs to be addressed.

At times, those underlying causes are actually outside influences which we subject our bodies too. They have little or nothing to do with food, but still have an obvious negative effect on our bodies. One such outside factor is swimming.

SWIMMING:
Swimming can also produce vaginal issues. Whether it is swimming in a naturally occurring body of water or a chlorinated swimming pool, they can both produce unwanted symptoms in the body.

Naturally occurring bodies of water have bacteria and other miniscule life forms present in the water that invade orifices when the body is submerged. The water is pushed into every open orifice and if the immune system is not sufficiently armed, an infection can develop.

Numerous cases of infection and illness have been reported at beaches due to the quantity of people swimming, some with sun tan lotion on which contaminates the water. Others have infections that are transmitted from their bodily tissues (as the water saturates internal tissues such as the vagina and anus) through the water to other people. Infections also arise from chlorinated pools.

Chlorine is harmful to the body. It kills the naturally-occurring good bacteria our bodies use to create balance and defense. It may kill other things in the water which are harmful, but it also kills the good bacteria which help balance our bodies. Because it has a drying effect, the natural lubricant that the vagina uses to trap and expunge invaders is destroyed, leaving the vagina basically dry and defenseless. It also kills the good bacteria on the skin which we need to live.

Because there are so many things which can negatively affect a women's intimate parts, organic douching is an inexpensive, holistic approach to counterbalancing the harmful effects that we have to deal with periodically.

There are many douches available that have profoundly positive effects on the body. Some douches are more effective for some women than others and some douches are more effective in addressing some problems than others. Any douche that is based on nature will work more effectively with immune system and may even boost the immune system. The douches discussed in this book are designed to work with the body to help restore balance and promote a healthy immune response.

The douches suggested in this book have been found to be effective, low cost and easy to use. This information is not given with the intent to diagnose a health issue. While the solutions presented here have shown that they work, they may not be applicable for every situation. Any implementation is the user's responsibility.

Chapter 2

The first douche is an organic douche which uses organic, plain Greek yogurt. Plain Greek yogurt is the most effective as it is gluten free and mostly sugar free. If a mild itching or discharge is present, many times using plain (not flavored) yogurt for 7 days will clear it up. The yogurt repopulates the healthy bacteria and flora which maintain a healthy intimate climate. It seems the most effective way to use Greek yogurt is to fill an (tampon) applicator with the yogurt and inject the yogurt lying on your back, much the same as inserting a tampon (complete directions below). As the yogurt warms in the body, it will liquefy, so pressing your knees downward towards the chest while lying on your back for as long as possible will help the yogurt sink to the bottom of the intimate cavity and coat the walls. Lying in this position helps the tissues absorb as much of the yogurt as possible. Immediately after injecting the yogurt, put some panties on to avoid wet spots. As the days go by, you will notice that less and less of the Greek yogurt is absorbed and more is being ejected from the body. This is a good sign as the body stops absorbing what it doesn't need.

To give the yeast a double whammy with the yogurt fix, eat the yogurt by itself with no additives or with honey to sweeten (no sugar to feed the yeast). This will attack the yeast in other parts of the body giving a much needed boost to the immune system. As the immune system is strengthened, it can rebalance itself easier and quicker.

Men can also use yogurt on their privates as yeast can exhibit itself with a partner.

DIRECTIONS:
When I first decided to try this, I had one problem: how do I inject the yogurt with no injector? While I have not seen applicators sold individually, there is a work around. Purchase the least expensive box of large plastic tampons that you can find. You will need 6 things: the empty tampon (plastic) tube, some tape or plastic wrap, a small paring knife or equivalent, a clean paper towel, a clean body towel and panties.

First, remove the tampon and separate the injector (top part) from the tampon holder (bottom part). Check the bottom of the injector (the part that pushes against the tampon). If there is an opening or it is hollow, put tape over the opening or use plastic wrap (must be thin) over the hole. If something other than tape is used, it needs to be about 2 inches long so there is enough to keep covering the hole as the plastic top moves through the applicator. If the end is left open and not covered, the yogurt will simply be pushed upward into the injector as the injector is pushed down in to the bottom (tampon holder) instead of the yogurt being pushed down the bottom into the vagina. The injector end is a tight fit into the tampon holder (bottom) piece. The injector end has to be squeezed, manipulated and maneuvered back into the bottom piece. This can be a little frustrating and messy, but it works.

Second, fill the bottom end (tampon end) with yogurt. I found using a small paring knife worked well as I could push the small knife tip into the bottom piece which pushes the yogurt further into the tube. Fill it completely. Once the bottom tube is filled, the injector needs to be fit back into the tube with any existing holes covered (tape or plastic wrap). When the injector is reinserted into the tube, some yogurt will be pushed out. Keep the pushed out yogurt as it can be rubbed on the outer area to kill any yeast there. Place the filled tube onto a new, clean paper towel.

Third, until you get the hang of it, put a towel down under your hips, lay on your back on the towel. Be sure to have a pair of panties handy. Rub the ejected yogurt that is on the tube end on the outer vaginal area. Then, inject the yogurt as deeply as possible into the vagina. Immediately after injection, remove the tube, put your panties on (stay on your back) and raise your knees to your chest. Stay in this position as long as possible. If you need to, move onto your side, but avoid sitting upright. You want the yogurt to remain in the cavity as long as possible.

This douche is effective if used once a day, at night, for up to 14 days.

Chapter 3

The second douche is a hydrogen peroxide mix. This remedy is handy for bacterial vaginosis or a simple bacterial infection. This mixture has been included because it is not an antibiotic or chemical product marketed for women's internal issues, but it is an antibacterial substance that works effectively to kill bacterial infections. Women can develop a bacterial infection in many ways: from a partner, not enough cleansing, bacteria from wiping the wrong way (should be front to back) and from unclean water sources (pools, lakes).

DIRECTIONS:
This simple douche works wonders. It starts to work immediately, is low cost and requires 5 items: hydrogen peroxide, clean water, a clean glass/container, bathtub and the tampon end (bottom end) of a tampon applicator.

First, get a clean glass. MAKE SURE THE GLASS AND WATER ARE CLEAN. Mix 1 cup hydrogen peroxide (a 3% peroxide solution) with 1 cup clean water. You can use any quantity of this mix if you need more, but the ratio of peroxide to water is 1:1.

Second, run hot water in the bathtub for about 2 minutes, keeping the drain open so the water goes down the drain. This will give you a warm spot to lie on versus a cold tub floor. You can also place a thick, fluffy towel on the tub floor and that will help protect from the cold. After the water has drained, lay in the tub on your back with your knees pressed towards your chest and your legs splayed open. This can be a little uncomfortable, but a rolled towel beneath your head/neck can help.

Third, your splayed legs will open the cavity into which the peroxide douche will be poured. Angle your hips upward as much as possible with your legs splayed open and pressed to your chest, open the feminine lips and pour the remedy over intimates until covered. Wait a minute for the mixture to be absorbed by the outer layers. Next, insert the bottom end of the plastic tampon applicator end into the feminine cavity as far as it will go. You want to ensure that you can pull it out, yet have it deep enough for the liquid to reach internally. Remember, keep your legs splayed and knees at chest level. The bottom end of the applicator inserted into the vagina opens the cavity and will ensure that the douche gets inside the cavity. Next, slowly pour the remaining liquid into the top of the bottom of the tampon holder as best as you can. You will feel it pour inside your body through the tampon tube. Keep pouring until you feel it coming back out or all the liquid has been used. You want to have enough liquid to feel it fill the cavity and start coming back out. You also want to use all of the remedy. So, if you didn't have enough liquid to feel it come back out, make a larger dose. Once the douche has been poured into the vaginal cavity, remove the tampon tube, but do not move. Wait for at least 5 minutes, lying on your back with your knees to your chest before moving. When you sit up, you will feel some of the liquid drain out.

NOTE: A douche bag can be used in lieu of the tampon, however, douche bags tend to develop mold which you cannot see because the inside of the bag and tube cannot be viewed. Mold can also develop inside the tube that connects the douche bag and applicator which is impossible to clean. I suggest the tampon method because a new tampon tube is sterilized and is disposable.

After 3 doses, the itching and discharge should subside, if not be completely gone. Sometimes a little irritation is experienced after a douche. Wait at least day one for the irritation to subside before douching again. Castor oil and coconut oil can be used in small amounts internally to ease irritation. They can be used on the days that douching does not occur.

This douche can be used every other day for 5 days, preferably at night. If irritation occurs, wait an extra day in between doses.

Chapter 4

The third douche is an organic douche. This remedy is a Grapefruit Seed extract mixture (not to be confused with Grapeseed). Grapefruit Seed extract addresses many issues including ear infections, gum disease, sinus infections, household cleaning as well as intimate imbalances. It is an antibacterial, antifungal and antiviral. It is derived from grapefruit. Because it is concentrated, only mere drops are needed to kill infection. The bottle will have the appropriate dosage for the area in which the extract is being applied.

DIRECTIONS:

This is another highly cost effective organic remedy which can be used for multiple purposes. This requires 5 items: Grapefruit Seed extract, a new tampon tube, clean water and a clean glass if using the tampon method. MAKE SURE THE GLASS AND WATER ARE CLEAN.

First, mix the Grapefruit Seed extract according to the directions with water. Be careful to use only the amount listed which is mere drops. Grapefruit Seed extract is concentrated. Only a little is needed and too much will cause irritation.

Second, run hot water in the bathtub for about 2 minutes, keeping the drain open so the water goes down the drain. This will give you a warm spot to lie on versus a cold tub floor or place a thick, fluffy towel on the tub floor. After the water has drained, lay in the tub on your back with your knees pressed towards your chest and your legs splayed open. This can be a little uncomfortable, but a rolled towel beneath your head/neck can help.

Third, your splayed legs will open the cavity into which the Grapefruit Seed douche will be poured. Angle your hips upward as much as possible, open the feminine lips and pour the remedy over the outer lips until they are covered. Wait a minute for the mixture to be absorbed by the outer layers. Next, insert the bottom end of the plastic tampon applicator end into the vagina as far as it will go. You want to ensure that you can pull it out, yet have it deep enough for the liquid to reach internally. Remember, keep your legs splayed and knees at chest level. The bottom end of the applicator inserted into the vagina opens the cavity and will ensure that the douche gets inside the cavity. Next, slowly pour the remaining liquid into the inserted tampon top as best as you can. You will feel it pour inside your body through the tampon tube. Keep pouring until you feel it coming back out or all the liquid has been used. You want to have enough liquid to feel it fill the cavity and start coming back out. You also want to use all of the remedy. So, if you didn't have enough liquid to feel it come back out, make a larger dose. Remove the tampon tube, but do not move. Wait for at least 5 minutes, lying on your back with your knees to your chest before moving. When you sit up, you will feel some of the liquid drain out.

NOTE: A douche bag can be used in lieu of the tampon, however, douche bags tend to develop mold which you cannot see because the inside of the bag and tube cannot be viewed. Mold can also develop inside the tube between the douche bag and applicator which is impossible to clean. I suggest the tampon method because a new tampon tube is sterilized and is disposable.

After 5 doses, the itching and discharge should subside, if not be completely gone. Sometimes a little irritation is experienced after a douche. Wait until the irritation subsides to douche again. Castor oil and coconut oil can be used in small amounts internally to ease irritation. They can be used on the days that douching does not occur.

Chapter 5

The fourth douche is a douche with a twist. This douche is organic, but involves extended douching by way of soaking. It is useful for internal stickiness, bacterial issues as well as yeast. This is a very gentle douche which means it works, but it is not as strong as other douches so it may take more time to affect a change. It is a great internal refresher. Even if there are no symptoms of anything, this douche can be used just to feel fresh.

DIRECTIONS:

This remedy is apple cider vinegar. There are 3 things needed: organic apple cider vinegar, water and a tub.

First, run a *warm* tub of water where the water level will be high enough to cover your hips when laying reclined on your back in the tub. Be sure the bathtub is clean prior to running the bathwater. A dirty bathtub will only waste your douche and exacerbate the issue. You will be encouraging water flow into the vagina and hot water can cause discomfort and damage to the delicate vaginal tissues. Add ½ cup of organic apple cider vinegar to the water and immerse the intimate cavity in the tub.

Second, lie as far back on your back with your legs splayed open. Sometimes it helps to heft a leg over the edge of the tub to open the cavity.

Third, rock your hips gently to start the water rolling. Using a hand can also produce small waves. Hold the outer feminine lips open with one hand while creating waves with other hand near the vaginal opening. This will allow greater access to the vaginal cavity while pushing the water inside. Do this for 15-30 minutes. Wait 24 hours and if there is no irritation, continue on for up to 7 days.

The apple cider vinegar will also soften your skin as well as balance the internals. You can combat an infection with a dual whammy similar to the yogurt. Take one tablespoon of apple cider vinegar internally every day. Some people can take it straight, others need to mix it in with 8 ounces of water. It will give you bitter beer face. It is very tart, but very effective.

Chapter 6

The fifth douche is another low cost, organic douche. It is also a soaking douche. What isn't used for the douche can be used for salad dressing, kitty smell, killing fire ant hills and making bleeding colors non-bleedable.

DIRECTIONS:
This douche is organic white vinegar. This follows the same method used in the other soaking douche. 3 things are needed: organic white vinegar, water and a tub.

First, run a warm tub of water where the water level will be high enough to cover your hips when laying reclined on your back in the tub. You will be encouraging water flow into the vaginal cavity and hot water can cause discomfort and damage. Add ½ cup of organic white vinegar to the water and immerse the vaginal cavity in the tub.

Second, lie as far back on your back as you can with your legs splayed open. Sometimes it helps to heft a leg over the edge of the tub to open the cavity.

Third, rock your hips gently to start the water rolling. Using a hand can also produce small waves. Hold the outer feminine lips open with one hand while creating waves with other hand near the vaginal opening. This will allow greater access to the vaginal cavity while pushing the water inside. Do this for 15-30 minutes. Wait 24 hours and if there is no irritation, continue on for up to 4 days.

White vinegar is stronger than apple cider vinegar so this douche remedy can be used up to 4 days as long as no irritation is present. Bear in mind that white vinegar also has a stronger drying effect on the vaginal tissues than apple cider vinegar.

Chapter 7

The sixth douche is a douche with a twist. This douche is organic, but involves extended douching by way of soaking. It is useful for internal stickiness, bacterial issues as well as yeast. This is a strong douche with strong antibacterial properties. It is a great internal refresher. Even if there are no symptoms of anything, this douche can be used just to feel fresh.

DIRECTIONS:
This remedy is tea tree oil. There are 3 things needed: organic tea tree oil, water and a tub.

First, run a warm tub of water where the water level will be high enough to cover your hips when laying reclined on your back in the tub. You will be encouraging water flow in the vaginal cavity and hot water can cause discomfort and damage. Add 10 drops of tea tree oil to the water and immerse the vaginal cavity in the tub.

Second, lie as far back on your back as you can with your legs splayed open. Sometimes it helps to heft a leg over the tub edge to open the cavity.

Third, rock your hips gently to start the water rolling. Using a hand can also produce small waves. Hold the outer feminine lips open with one hand while creating waves with other hand near the vaginal opening. This will allow greater access to the intimate cavity while pushing the water inside. Do this for 15-30 minutes. Wait 24 hours and if there is no irritation, continue on for up to 7 days.

Chapter 8

Organic douches are a low cost, effective remedy for many vaginal discomforts. Unlike antibiotics, organic remedies work with the body and immune system to fight infection and restore natural balance. It has been speculated that the body builds immunity to antibiotics because they don't work hand in hand with the body's natural fighting abilities. Antibiotics have a tendency to lower the immune system while fighting whatever bug the antibiotic is scripted for. This causes imbalance in other areas which leaves the body open to more issues. I know someone who became pregnant because she was taking antibiotics and it made her birth control null and void. That was an expensive antibiotic!

Why use a product that lowers the immune system instead of one that works with the immune system and may even boost the immune system?

It seems a ludicrous question, yet many people are unaware of just how powerful and effective natural remedies are. This is one of the reasons I decided to write this book. Some people are also unaware that costly doctor visits and exorbitant prescriptions are not always the answer. Sometimes, they aren't needed at all. Just a little bit of information goes a long way just like a little bit of nature goes a long way.

Try these organic, low cost remedies for yourself. If they help you, please invite your friends to buy this book. 10% of all proceeds are donated to charity. The rest is used to promote healthier alternatives via new books for you.

Also, the more reviews the book receives on Amazon, the more people will be reached with this great information so please feel free to leave a review!

Thank you for purchasing this book. For more organic, low cost lifestyle tips, visit www.digitalquill.top.

Bonus Information:

A woman I helped with chronic ear infections had an awesome testimonial. She had been battling chronic ear infections for years. Because the antibiotics had ceased to work, they put tubes in her ears and told her she would have to have surgery. After suggesting the organic approach, she tried it before undergoing an expensive surgery. Following the directions, her ears began to unclog, then they began to drain. This happened in only 3 days of using the Grapefruit Seed extract versus years of antibiotics. After two weeks, the infection had cleared up and neither the tubes nor the surgery were needed. Eventually, her infections stopped altogether which was my experience also because Grapefruit Seed helps to build the immune system.

I had an issue with chronic sinus infections. Eventually, after a year and a half of emergency room visits, they told me they couldn't help me because they had given me dual rounds of the most current antibiotic at double the normal length and I was still not cured. I knew there had to be a solution so I went to the health food store and was introduced to Grapefruit Seed extract. It took a couple of weeks to wipe out that infection, but each infection got shorter and easier to kill. A year later, I had no more sinus infections. Even after moving to different regions, when I experienced a twinge, I would use the Grapefruit Seed and the sinus headaches stopped and the infection cleared up. I haven't had a sinus infection in years.

What are your health goals?

Who are you listening to for health advice?

Are you taking ownership of your health?

How can you improve your health and vitality?

Is your health all that you want it to be?

Are you *ready* to live a happier, healthier life?